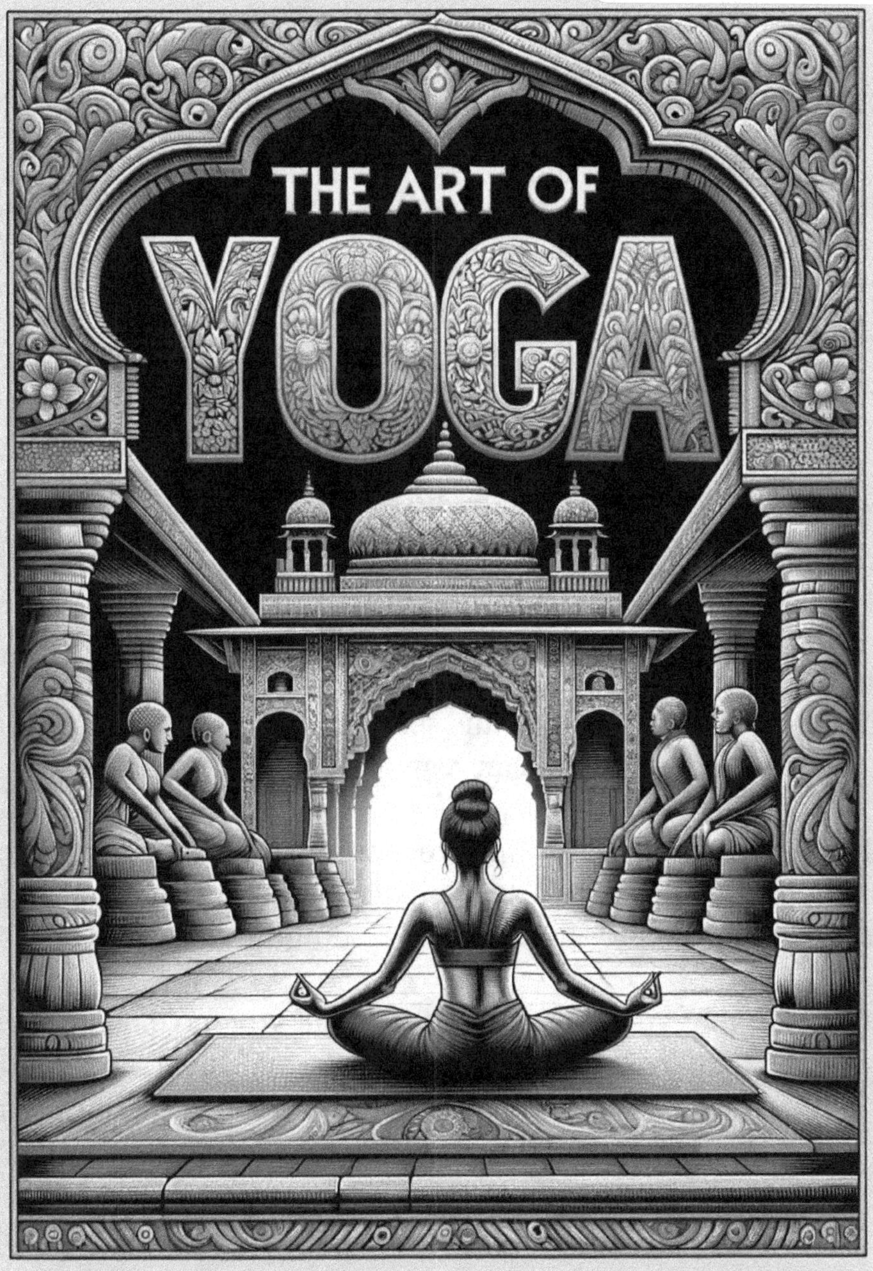

THE ART OF YOGA

The practice of yoga, sometimes known as the "magic word," has led people worldwide to improve physical health, mental tranquility, and even financial success. The practice of yoga has the potential to completely change a person's life and transport them to a mind-blowing state of peace and tranquility. Few people are familiar with the capabilities of yoga and the asanas that are suggested by this one-of-a-kind healing science.

There are also a lot of people who have preconceived beliefs about yoga based on what they have seen or heard, even though they have no idea what yoga is. It is crucial to have a solid understanding of what yoga is and its foundational principles before practicing it. This will ensure that the advantages of yoga penetrate deep into your being and that you are able to apply this science in the most effective manner possible so that you can reap the greatest rewards.

 What are some of the first things that come to mind when you hear the word "Yoga"? You have seen pictures of ladies striking what appear to be impossible stances at some point in your life.

If you believe that yoga is solely about what you have heard from other people, then you may only have a cursory understanding of this remarkable subject. However, there is a significant amount of more information to learn about yoga, and doing so requires a significant amount of time and effort.

This book will concentrate its attention primarily on the following facets of yoga:

- The justifications for why you should engage in yoga practice

- The advantages of participating in yoga practices

- Yoga positions and some of the most prevalent errors that should be avoided

It is my firm conviction that reading this e-book will present you with the solutions to all of the problems that you might experience in relation to practicing yoga. You will be presented with the most important yoga positions that can be done by everyone without much difficulty.

Charles van Veen

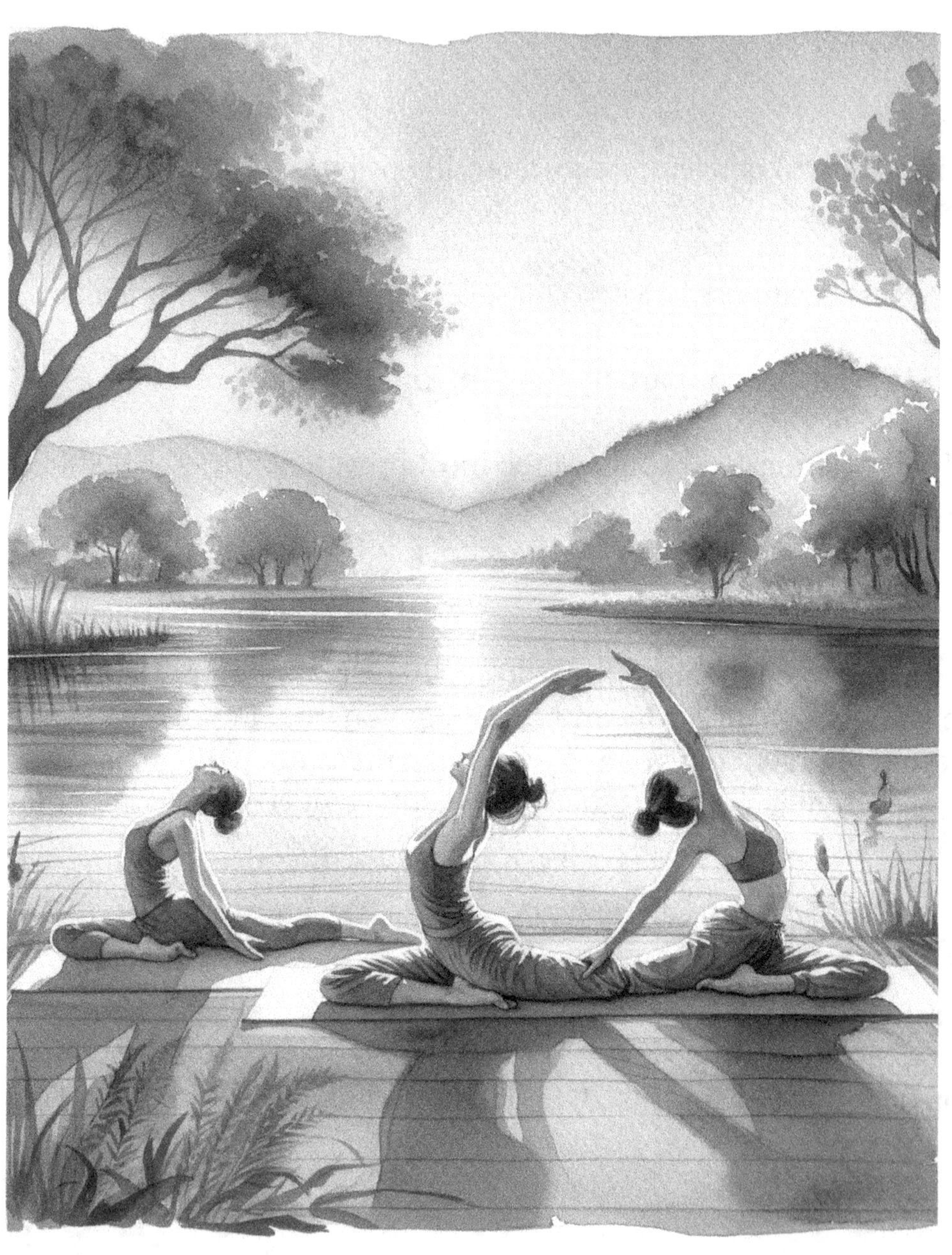

There are seven basic styles of yoga, and they are called Hatha, Vinyasa, Power, Ashtanga, and Iyengar yoga, respectively.

The most widely practised and accessible style of yoga is Hatha Yoga,

Hatha brings together a variety of different breathing practices and fundamental movement sequences.

Vinyasa yoga is distinguished by its use of a series of positions that flow seamlessly into one another.

Ashtanga yoga is like Vinyasa yoga in that it combines many postures that transition fluidly into one another; however, the poses in Ashtanga yoga also use specialized breathing methods.

Power yoga is an aggressive kind of yoga that is designed to strengthen muscles rapidly.

Bikram is a style of yoga that consists of 26 different postures that are practised in extremely hot temperatures.

Iyengar yoga makes use of props, such as blocks and chairs, to help align the body in the appropriate position during the practice.

In this book, we will concentrate mostly on Hatha Yoga, which is the foundational style of yoga. If you have already set routines and successfully incorporated yoga into your life, you may be a committed practitioner of yoga.

Yoga is a flexible kind of exercise that can be adapted to suit any lifestyle. It is possible to put its principles into effect virtually anywhere, whether at home when travelling by air, or while working at a desk.

Because yoga does not call for the use of any specialized apparatus, it is simple to continue your regular practice even when you are away from home, which is one of its many advantages.

You can still incorporate yoga into your daily routine, even if your life is busy, even if it is only for five minutes at a time. All it takes is a little bit of dedication and commitment.

If you currently have a regular workout program, adding yoga to either the beginning or the conclusion of it is a simple and straightforward process.

It does not matter if your schedule is always the same or always changing; you can still practice yoga on a regular basis. You can always find space for yoga, regardless of where you live, be it in a mountain or by the beach, in a one-bedroom apartment or a palace with twenty bedrooms.

To put it another way, there is no justification for excluding it from your life, especially considering the multiple advantages it possesses.

Why don't you just try it?

If you already have a set pattern for your workouts, adding a single yoga pose to your cool-down routine is a simple and straightforward process. Before moving on to anything else, try practicing only one pose for several days in a row.

This allows your body the time it needs to adjust to the new configuration and understand its procedure, which is often more difficult than it seems on the surface.

The "when" and "where" of yoga are irrelevant as long as the practice is maintained on a regular basis.

The beneficial effects of yoga can only be attained via regular practice. To see the obvious effects of their yoga practice, many people find that it is beneficial to wake up thirty minutes earlier than they would normally to begin their practice.

Doing yoga first thing in the morning is a fantastic way to start the day. A lot of people swear by yoga as a nighttime practice because they believe it makes it simpler for them to nod off. You do not have time to wake up thirty minutes earlier, do you? You can also practice yoga at work if the conditions there are conducive to it.

A sizable number of the positions can be conducted while seated on a chair. While you are waiting in line or standing in line, you can execute other people. The sole rule is that you should not practice yoga for at least a couple of hours after you have eaten.

If you want to make it simpler for yourself to practice yoga whenever and whenever the opportunity arises, I suggest having a yoga mat and a set of comfortable workout clothing in your car. This will make it easier for you to do yoga. It is hard to say when you might need that information.

Even though you can practice yoga pretty much anywhere, my suggestion is that you designate a calm and cosy area of your home just for yoga practice.

One of my friends was extraordinarily lucky to have an extra room in her house, which she subsequently dedicated to the practice of yoga.

The space, which she referred to as "The Yoga Room," was carpeted, the walls were clear of clutter, and the room contained only the things she needed for her yoga practice.

It was spotless, open, invigorating, and soothing, in other words, the ideal environment for yoga. Even if you do not have enough room to devote a whole room to yoga, you may at least clear off a section of a room to use for the practice. It is best to do this near a wall, as you may occasionally need to lean against it for support.

Creating a strategy is the next stage after that. It is essential that you ease into the practice of yoga if you are just starting out with this practice and yoga in general.

Your body needs a period to gradually adapt to the changes that you are making to it. While this is going on, your physical self needs to go through the motions of yoga on a consistent basis for you to start reaping the benefits of yoga in all three realms of your being (body, mind, and spirit).

If you allow yourself five minutes every day, you can ease into yoga by practicing one or two positions. This is a wonderful way to get started with yoga. You only need to set aside five minutes at the beginning.

Integrate it into one of the routines you already have. For instance, if you have a specific ritual that you follow to begin each day, adding five minutes of yoga to the end of that process can assist you in decluttering your thoughts and getting your body and mind ready for action.

On the other hand, if you have a routine that you always complete before you go to bed (and if you don't, I strongly suggest that you start), doing five minutes of yoga will help you relax and can prepare both your mind and body for a restful night's sleep. If you do not have a routine, I highly recommend that you start one.

Begin with one or two positions that seem comfortable to you.
After a few weeks, you should experiment with a new stance or two.
When you start to experience the benefits of yoga, such as increased
alertness and flexibility, among other things, feel free to extend the
amount of time you spend practicing yoga to 10 minutes per day or
even longer.

When you have developed your yoga practice to the point that you
can do sessions lasting 20 or 30 minutes at a time, you should think
about devoting a certain time to your yoga routine.

You are welcome to continue practicing yoga either at the beginning
or the end of your day; but, if you discover that it makes your
mornings or nights feel rushed, you are welcome to try practicing it at
other times of the day.

I recommend that you keep using one or two yoga postures to assist
you in waking up and to assist you in preparing for sleep. At the same
time, I suggest that you allow yourself at least three defined blocks of
time each week to devote to a more extended practice of yoga.

Yoga has been shown to have a variety of health benefits, some of which include the reduction of physical and mental stress, a slowed rate of ageing, an improvement in mood, along with relaxation and a sense of calm.

On the other hand, newcomers to yoga frequently, and typically because of their excessive excitement, make some errors in their comprehension of and approach to the practice of yoga, and they attempt the poses without the benefit of adequate instruction.

Not only inexperienced yogis but also more seasoned practitioners, make errors in their form when working through the various yoga postures. They would undoubtedly profit from some fine-tuning and being aware of the typical blunders that people make when practicing yoga.

1. Putting in excessive effort

It has been observed that most people are aware of themselves when they are trying to push themselves beyond their capabilities, but they still like doing it.

This is the case because the phrase "No pain, no gain" comes to mind whenever we think of physical activity. Even when we work out at a gym, we are not happy with the session until our muscles start to groan in protest. Only then do we consider the activity a success.

But yoga is the complete antithesis of it. If you feel discomfort in your muscles when you are working out, it is a warning sign that you are heading in the direction of an injury or muscle strain. Asanas in yoga should never be painful for the student.

Awareness is the focus of yoga. The key is to pay attention to the hints that are being sent to you by your body, and then act in accordance with those hints. Therefore, you need to ease up on it if it starts to get uncomfortable.

2. Putting oneself in other people's shoes

When you begin practicing yoga, whether at home or in a class, you will inevitably come across some incredibly flexible yogis or their images who seem to effortlessly master each pose.

Their adaptability is sure to make you feel inadequate in comparison, and you secretly want to one day achieve their level. Having said that, attaining it is not a simple task.

It requires a lot of practice over many years. When you compare yourself to others, all you will accomplish is to give yourself a great deal of frustration, and you may wind up persuading yourself that yoga is not for you.

Therefore, you need to resist the temptation to judge yourself harshly by drawing comparisons between yourself and more experienced yogis.

3. Making the mistake of practicing at the incorrect spot

If you want to participate in yoga lessons, where do you believe you will have the most success? You would probably want to be at the front, wouldn't you? Is that right? Not true! Go to the back of the room if you want to arrange your mat in the most advantageous position.

It is not necessary to be near the front of the room to view the instructor because, in most cases, he or she will be roaming about the room and assisting people in correcting their poses.

You might also try the row that comes before the very last one. You might need to turn around and face the back of the room for certain maneuvers.

Therefore, positioning yourself in the row before the very last one will ensure that you will always have someone to follow without requiring you to break your form to look to the side.

4. Performing yoga postures while one has a full stomach

When practicing yoga positions, you should never do so while you are full. When you have food in your stomach, it can make some of the positions difficult to perform.

In addition, because your blood supply is being diverted to your digestive organs, it is possible that your muscles may not receive the adequate amount of energy that is required for productive exercise.

We are all in agreement that the food we eat acts as fuel for our bodies. To get the most out of this fuel, however, you need to eat approximately an hour before your workout and limit the amount of food you consume during each meal.

Before attempting your first posture, doing so will ensure that the blood has sufficient time to digest the food, collect the stimulating nutrients, and then transfer them onto the muscles.

5. Maintaining a daily practice of asanas

Building muscle is one of the benefits of practicing yoga. However, you need to allow your muscles some time to recover from the microscopic tears that are caused by each workout, particularly in the beginning of your exercise routine.

Therefore, if you are just beginning out with yoga, it is recommended that you practice once every other day; otherwise, your muscles will become fatigued.

6. Not sufficiently warming up the muscles

The constant feeling of being rushed for time is an inevitable aspect of our lifestyle. Because of the limited amount of time, you might feel tempted to skip the warm-up exercises and jump right into a difficult position.

However, doing so will unquestionably raise the possibility of you getting hurt. It is imperative that you engage in some form of stretching for at least five minutes to warm up your body to the point where it can more readily assume the more difficult poses.

7. Failure to properly cool down after exercise

Each yoga session begins with a warm-up, and it concludes with a cool-down. Both steps are necessary for optimal results.

Before beginning your next workout, it is imperative that you engage in a cool-down session that lasts for at least ten minutes. This will assist in the recovery and repair of your muscles and ligaments.

This can also help you avoid fainting or dizziness, which can occur due to blood pooling in the legs during standing postures. This is because standing postures cause blood to pool in the legs.

Not only can anyone practice yoga as long as they have a mat, but yoga can also be done anywhere, making it accessible to individuals of all ages, stages of life, and physical abilities.

Pregnant women, persons with limited mobility, and seniors can all benefit from practicing yoga. However, being able to perform certain yoga poses does not guarantee that you are performing them correctly or that you are making the most of the time and effort that you are investing in your yoga practice.

When you practice yoga, it is essential to be mindful of your shortcomings and try to improve them so that both your awareness and your form are not negatively impacted.

If you can avoid making these typical errors that beginners make, you will be able to get the most out of your workouts and have a lower chance of getting hurt. Also, keep in mind that yoga is a continual practice, and that your objective should be to continuously develop to reach perfection.

Pose of the Half Wheel

If you partied over the weekend, Half Wheel Pose is an excellent beginner posture for you to practice when you get back to work on Monday morning. Even if you have not done yoga before, beginning your practice with this position is a terrific way to get started.

The Half Wheel Pose is excellent for aiding digestion. Indigestion, as you are well known, is the underlying cause of several different conditions. Indigestion and other digestive issues are symptoms that can be brought into the workplace from overindulging in food over the weekend. Begin with the Half Wheel Pose before moving on to the next pose.

How it works:

Maintain a straight stance with your feet together and your hands resting by your sides.

As you raise your arms above your head and back, take a deep breath in.

Increase the depth of your bend as much as you can.

Hold the position for a total of twenty seconds.

You can make bending over easier by positioning your chair so that it is behind you and grabbing the back of the chair as you do so.

Advantages:

The Half Wheel Pose is beneficial for digestive health.

It relieves discomfort in the back while also toning the back muscles.

Your lung capacity will increase in addition to your lung strength.

This stance is excellent for improving heart function and regulating blood pressure.

Important things to keep in mind:

Avoid bending your knees in any way. Maintain a straight elbow position while you bend your arms behind your back.

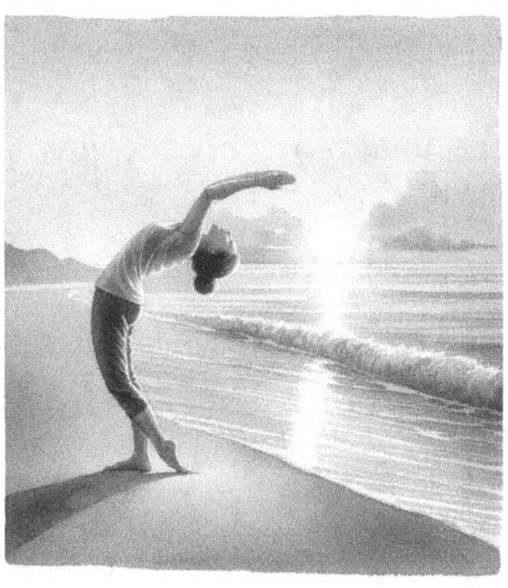

While Standing Perform a Forward Bend

One of the most beneficial poses for stretching your entire body is the standing forward bend. Your muscles are toned all over your body.

How it works:

Maintain a straight stance and place your hands on your sides.

Raise your hands over your head and hold them there. Put the palms of your hands facing one another.

As you bend forward and reach for the ground with your fingers, take a few deep breaths in through your nose.

Put your hands down by your feet, palms facing outward. You can also put your palms behind your legs and hold them, or you can just position them behind your legs.

Move your face so that it is in closer proximity to your legs. You should strive to bring your forehead down to touch both of your legs.

Hold the position for a total of twenty seconds.

Advantages:

Pain in the neck can be relieved with a standing forward bend.

It is helpful for conditions related to sciatica.

The position is relaxing and helps relieve stress.

It encourages more blood to flow to the brain and calms the mind at the same time.

Important things to keep in mind:

When you are attempting to reach the ground, you should not bend your knees.

Shoulders tend to be held in a rigid position by many beginners. Concentrate on your entire body and make sure that each and every aspect of it is completely at ease.

It is important to note that individuals who have high blood pressure or vision problems should not perform the Standing Forward Bend.

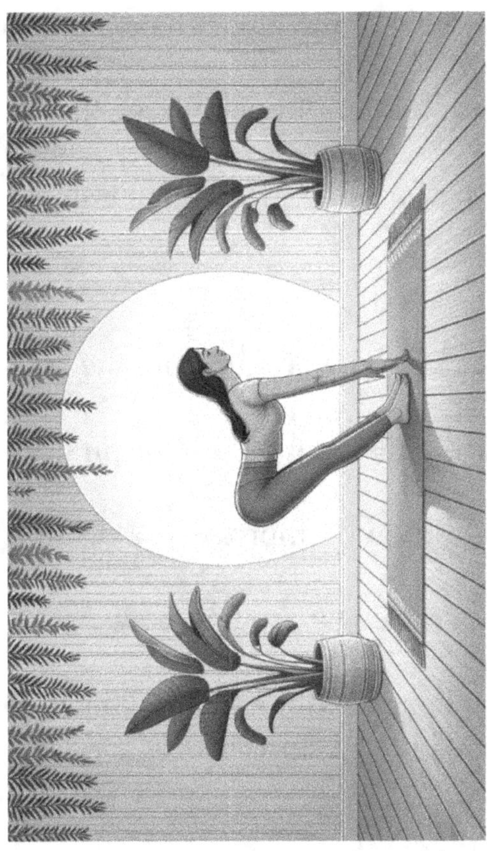

Pose of the Half Wheel of the Waist

Increase your hip range of motion by practicing the Half Waist Wheel Pose. Because you do not usually bend to the side like this very often, holding this position will help your hips become more flexible. Additionally, it improves the strength of your back.

How it works:

Maintain this stance with your feet touching. Raise both hands over your head and bring the palms of your hands into contact with one another.

Draw air in.

As you bend to the right at the hip, exhale as you move your body.

Hold the position for a total of twenty seconds.

On the other side, perform the identical actions.

Advantages:

Your lungs will get a good workout from the Half Waist Wheel Pose.

It is useful for treating disorders of the respiratory system.

Your level of flexibility will improve as a result.

This position helps reduce fat around the waist.

Important things to keep in mind: While you are holding this stance, you should not bend either backwards or forward.

Note:
Those who have experienced hip damage should refrain from holding this stance.

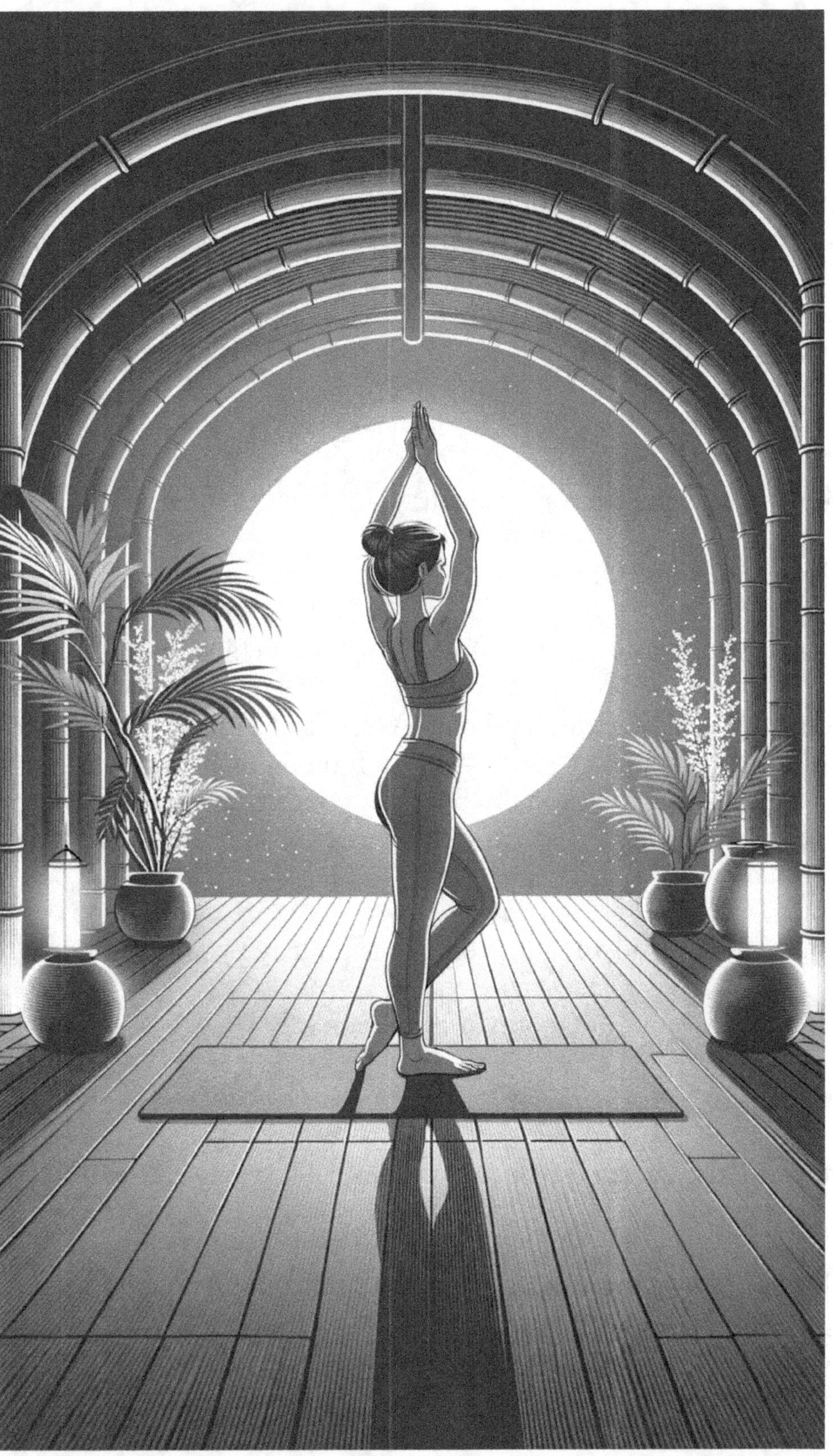

Forward Bend While Seated

One of the most effective poses for boosting your energy is the seated forward bend. Your shoulders, upper back, and neck will all feel better because of the stress relief. As soon as you start feeling the effects of work on your back and neck, the second day on the job is the absolute earliest you should attempt this stance. This pose is one of many that you are free to do on any day of the week.

How it works:

Take a seat on the rim of the chair.

Raise your hands over your head and hold them there.

Release your breath and lean forward from the hips.

Bring your arms forward and place them next to your feet in a side-by-side position. You could either position them in front of your feet, or you could put your arms in between your knees and lay your palms up beneath the chair's legs. Another option is to position them behind your back.

Bring your head down, and let the tension leave your shoulders.

Hold this position for a count of 15 seconds.

Advantages:

Stretching the spine and the neck is the goal of the seated forward bend.

It does this by improving the function of the abdominal organs.

The posture has a calming effect on the mind.

Important things to keep in mind:

Put your upper body, including your chest and abdomen, on top of your thighs. You should try to stretch your spine as much as you can.

Note: People who have hypertension should position their head so that it is higher than their heart.

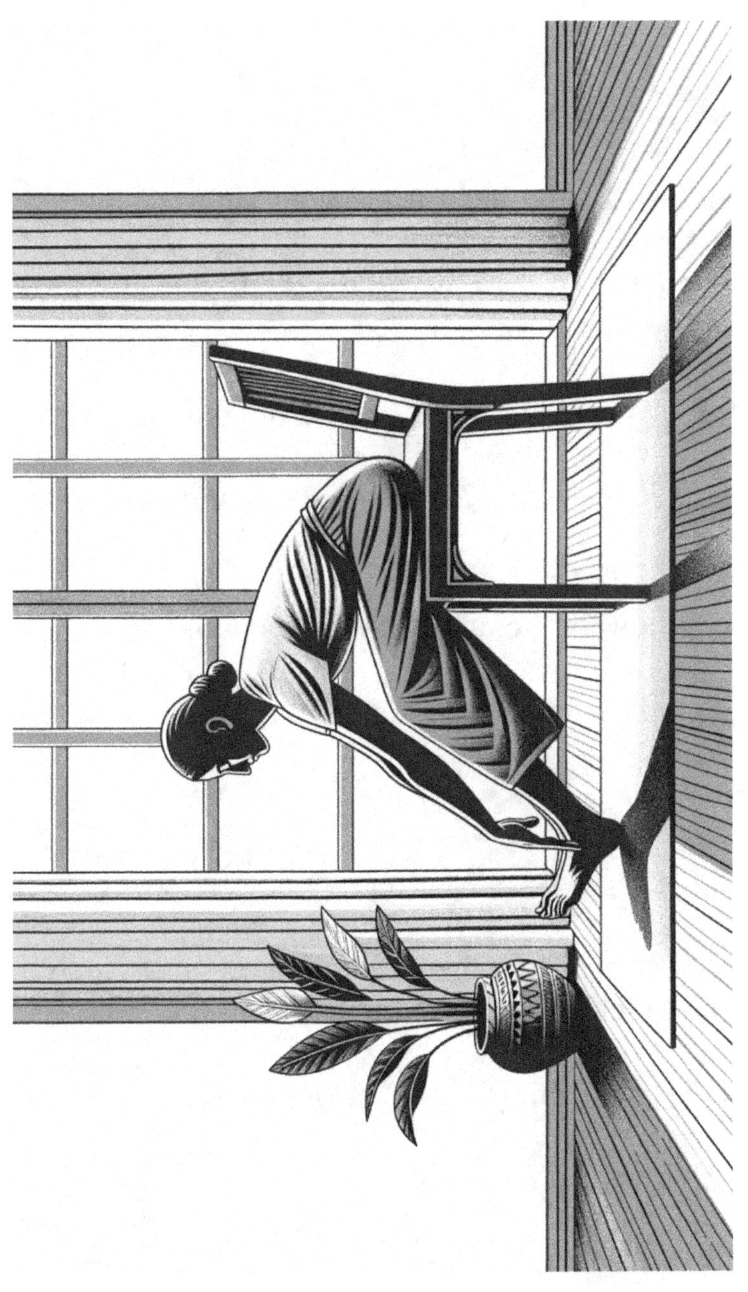

Twist While Seated in a Chair

Seated Chair Twist is yet another stunning and beneficial yoga stance that can be performed from the convenience of a chair. This pose tones your back and hips.

How it works:

Please make yourself comfortable in the chair.

Take a deep breath out, then turn to your right.

Bring your left arm over to the right side of your body and rest it on the outside of your right thigh.

Put the palm of your right hand behind the buttock on your right side.

You should face the right side of the room and peek over your right shoulder.

Hold this position for a count of thirty seconds.

On the other side, perform the identical actions.

Advantages:

The Seated Chair Twist is an effective back exercise.

It does this by stimulating the abdominal organs, which in turn improves the function of those organs.

It helps increase flexibility in the hips.

It relieves discomfort in the neck.

Important things to keep in mind:

Do not lift your feet off the ground. It is imperative that the lower section of the body not be turned.

Note: Individuals who are experiencing significant neck pain should look directly ahead rather than glancing over their shoulder.

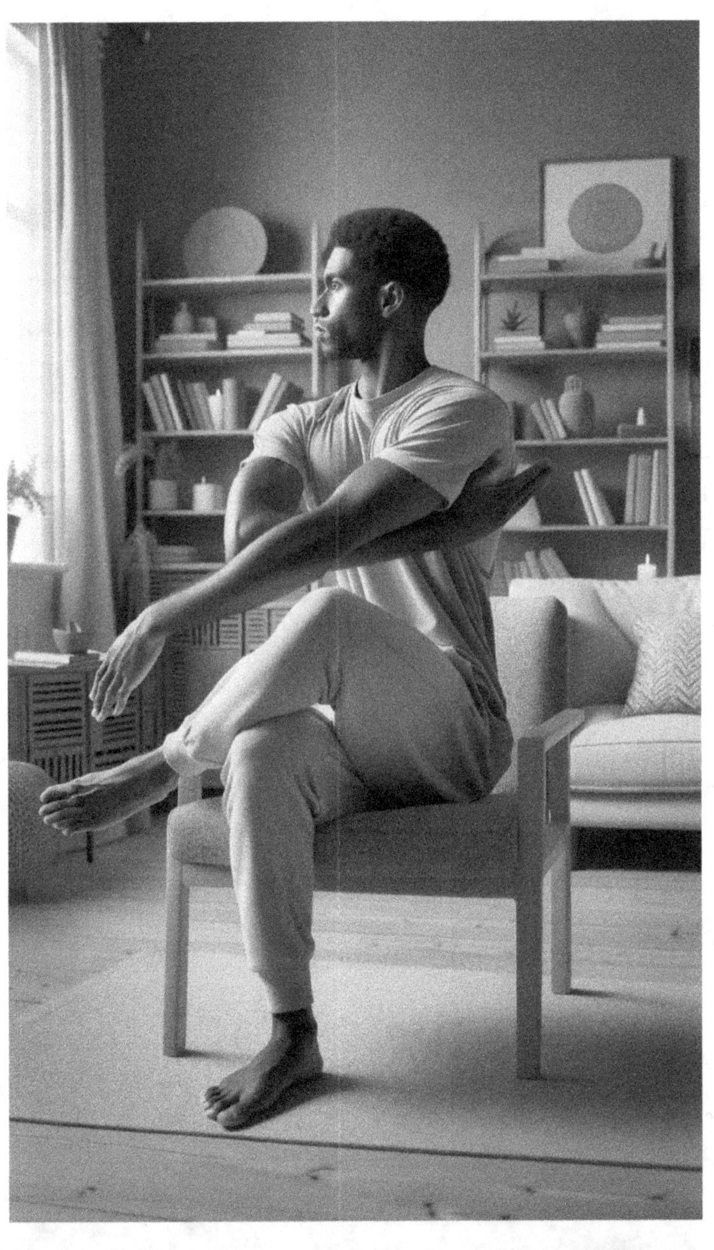

Backbend While Seated

The seated back bend helps to relax the muscles in your back and neck, which can help you feel much better overall. If you spend most of your time at work sitting at a desk, the Seated Back Bend can be an excellent approach to provide your back with the relief and attention it so desperately needs.

How it works:

Place your bottom in the middle of the chair's seat.

Bring your hands around to the back of your seat so that you can grab the armrests behind you. You also have the option of holding the lower portion of the backrest on either side of the chair.

Take a deep breath in and lean forward from the hips as you exhale. While doing so, tilt your head back as far as it comfortably can go. Arch your back.

Hold the position for a total of twenty seconds.

Advantages:

The Seated Back Bend is effective at relieving pain in the back.

The muscles in the shoulder are relieved as a result.

It is helpful for relieving pain in the neck.

The asana helps to increase one's lung capacity.

Important things to keep in mind:

Always keep your heels down. Be sure to keep both of your feet firmly planted on the floor. Maintain a straight position of the elbows. If you notice that your shoulders are rounded forward, shift your seating position such that they are parallel to the floor. This will allow your shoulders to relax.

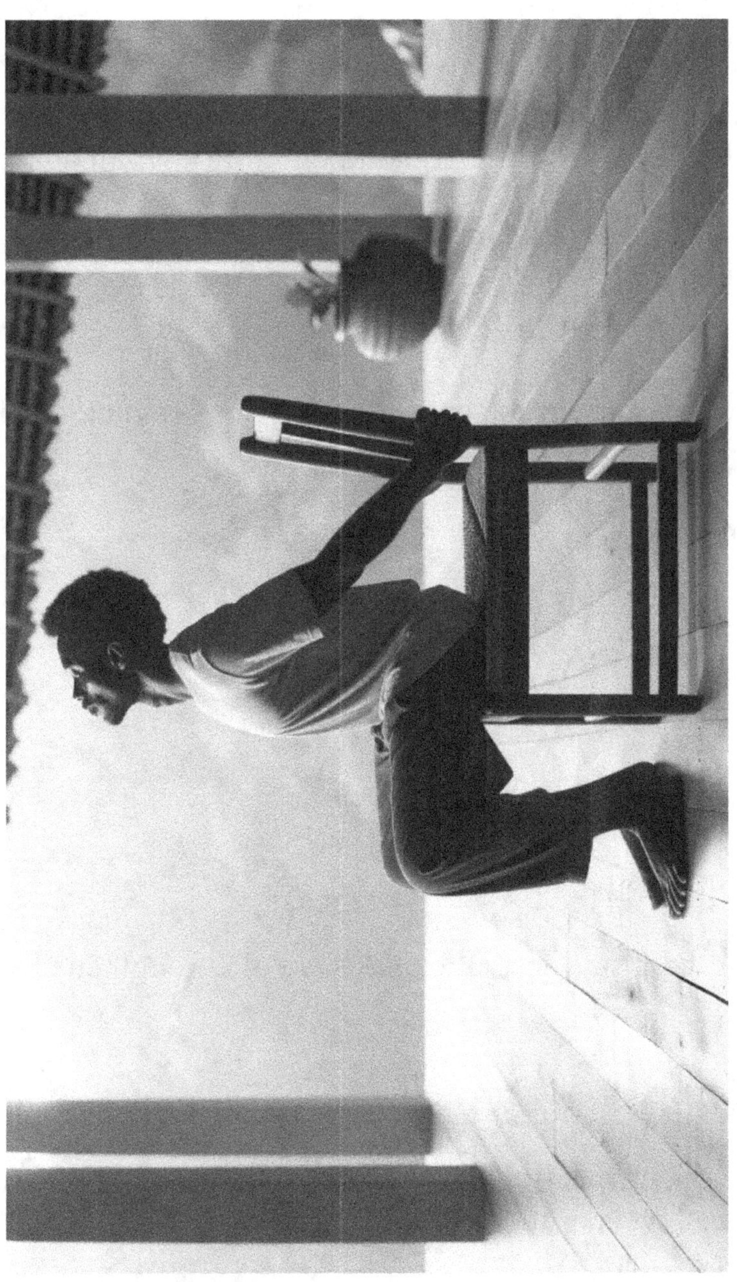

Pose a la chaise.

Although it is called the Chair position, the most interesting and difficult part of the position is that you are supposed to sit in a chair that does not actually exist. The Chair Pose is excellent for strengthening the immune system. The procedure is as follows.

How it works:

Maintain a straight stance with your hands resting at your sides. Keep a spacing between your feet equal to one foot's width apart.

Raise your hands in front of you and bring them to the same height as your shoulders. You can try reaching your hands over your head in a variety of diverse ways.

As you lower your butt to achieve sitting posture on an imaginary chair, exhale slowly as you do so.

Maintain the position for one full minute.

Advantages:

The Chair Pose is good for your immunity.

It strengthens both your back and spine.

It gives your legs more strength.

Hip flexors, calf muscles, and ankles are all strengthened by holding this pose.

It is beneficial to the heart's health.

It does this by stimulating the abdominal organs and boosting the performance levels of those organs.

Important things to keep in mind:

Do not lean forward an excessive amount. Make an effort to bring your butt down as far as you can without moving too far forward.

Caution: Those who suffer from low blood pressure or insomnia should not attempt to practice the chair pose.

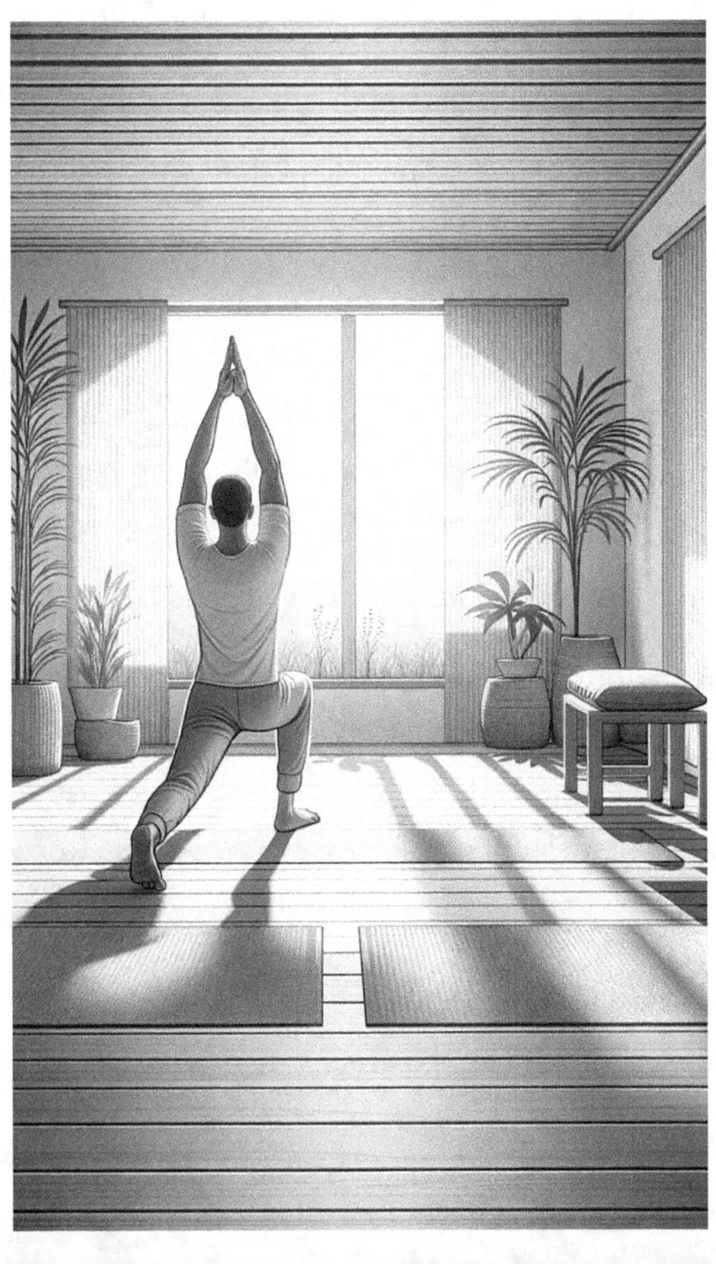

Pose with a Turning Chair

The Revolved Chair Pose is a modification of the Chair Pose that can assist you in bringing out the best in yourself. The more you practice the position, the more you will see the challenger in you.

How it works:

Maintain an upright stance with your feet touching.

As you bow your knees and lower your butt, let out an exhalation.

Put your kneecaps in a position where they are directly above your toes.

Turn your right hip to the right side and bring your left arm around to the right side of your body.

In the position known as the "salutation," bring both palms together. It is recommended that you position the elbow of your left hand so that it is on the outside of the right knee.

Hold this position for a count of thirty seconds.

On the other side, perform the identical actions.

Advantages:

The hip flexors are strengthened by practice of the Revolved Chair Pose.

Calf muscles are stretched out as a result.

It does this by stimulating the organs in your abdominal cavity.

It helps the digestive process.

The position encourages detoxification in the body.

Your upper back and shoulders will become toned because of this.

It has a beneficial effect on lung function.

Important things to keep in mind:

When attempting to maintain balance in the position, many people make the mistake of spreading their feet apart.

Note: Those who struggle with insomnia should refrain from striking the stance altogether. Avoiding the Revolved Chair Pose is also recommended for individuals who have a low blood pressure reading.

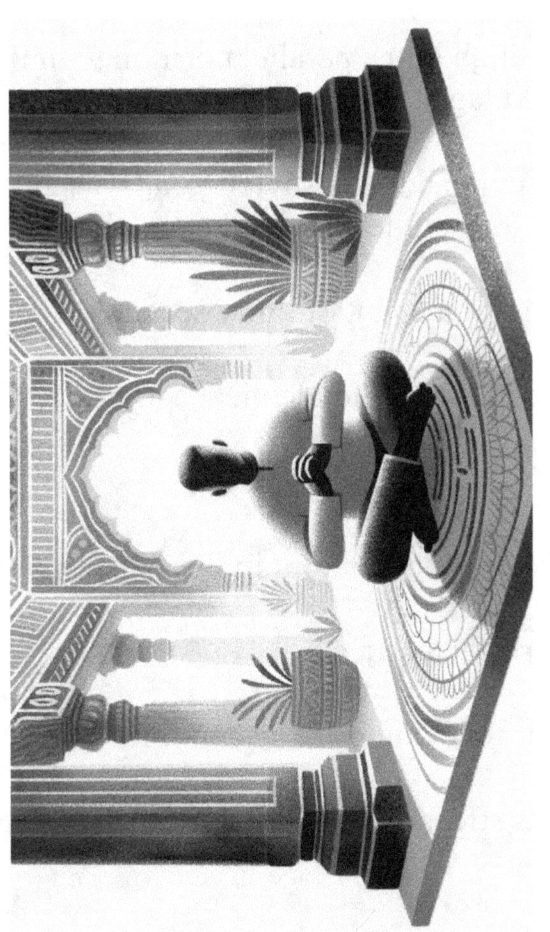

Position of the Warrior II

Your legs will get a good workout in the Warrior II Pose. This is a splendid example of a stance that requires you to maintain your balance.

How it works:

Maintain a straight stance with around two meters (about four feet) of space between your feet.

You should now rotate your right foot so that it is pointing in a direction that is 90 degrees to the right.

Bring your right thigh into a parallel position with the floor by bending your right leg at the knee.

Take a deep breath in and then stretch your arms out to the side. Place the hands so that they are level with the shoulders.

Hold this position for a count of thirty seconds.

On the other side, perform the identical actions.

Advantages:

Your legs will get a good workout in the Warrior II Pose.

It makes one more balanced.

It is beneficial for relieving back discomfort.

It has a beneficial effect on lung capacity.

Important things to keep in mind:

You can achieve the stance either with or without the chair.

It is important to note that individuals who have hypertension should not practice this position.

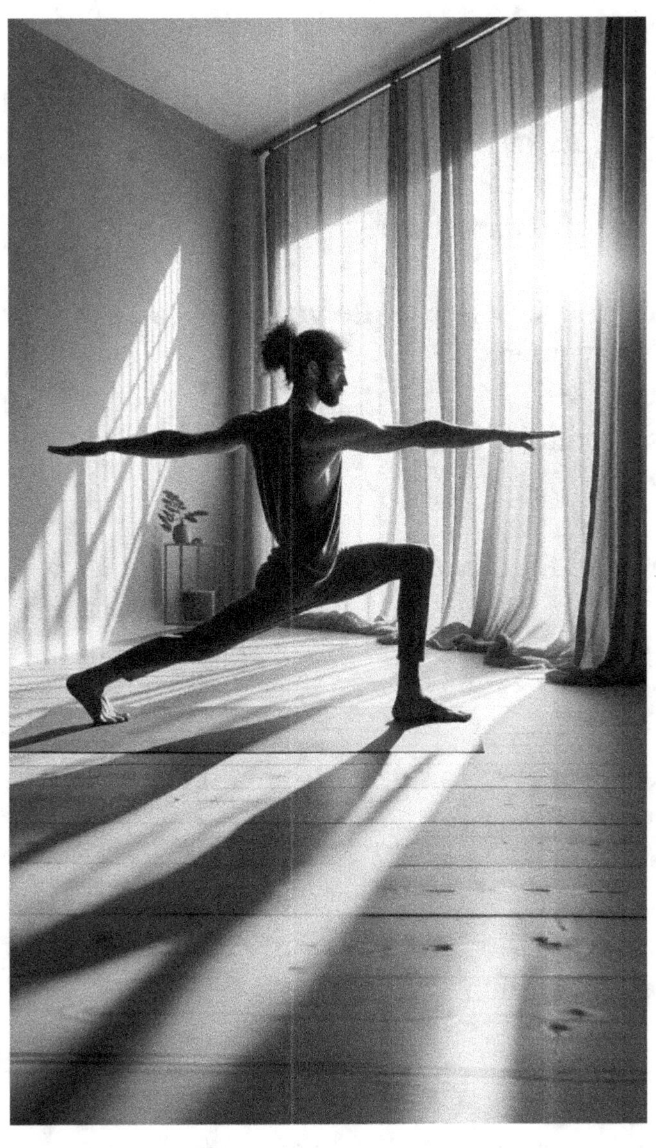

Pose à la Montagne.

Although it might not look like it, Mountain posture demands quite a bit of concentration on your part to be performed correctly. If you want to get the most out of this posture, you need to pay attention. In addition to that, it offers significant advantages to one's health. Given the amount of stress that you have been going through over the course of the week, the position is going to be of exceptional use to you.

How it works:

Place your hands on your knees and sit on the chair so that your back is completely straight.

Take a deep breath in and then stretch your arms out to the side.

As you exhale and slowly elevate your arms above your head, continue the movement.

Your fingers should be interlocked, and your palms should be facing upward.

Hold this position for a count of thirty seconds.

Advantages:

Your spine will benefit from the Mountain Pose's ability to lengthen and extend it.

It strengthens your neck, shoulders, and back all at the same time.

This exercise will stretch your hips.

It has a beneficial effect on lung capacity.

This pose is fantastic for putting all the joints in your arms to work.

Important things to keep in mind:

Always remember to keep a straight spine. The correct position for your hands is straight above your head.

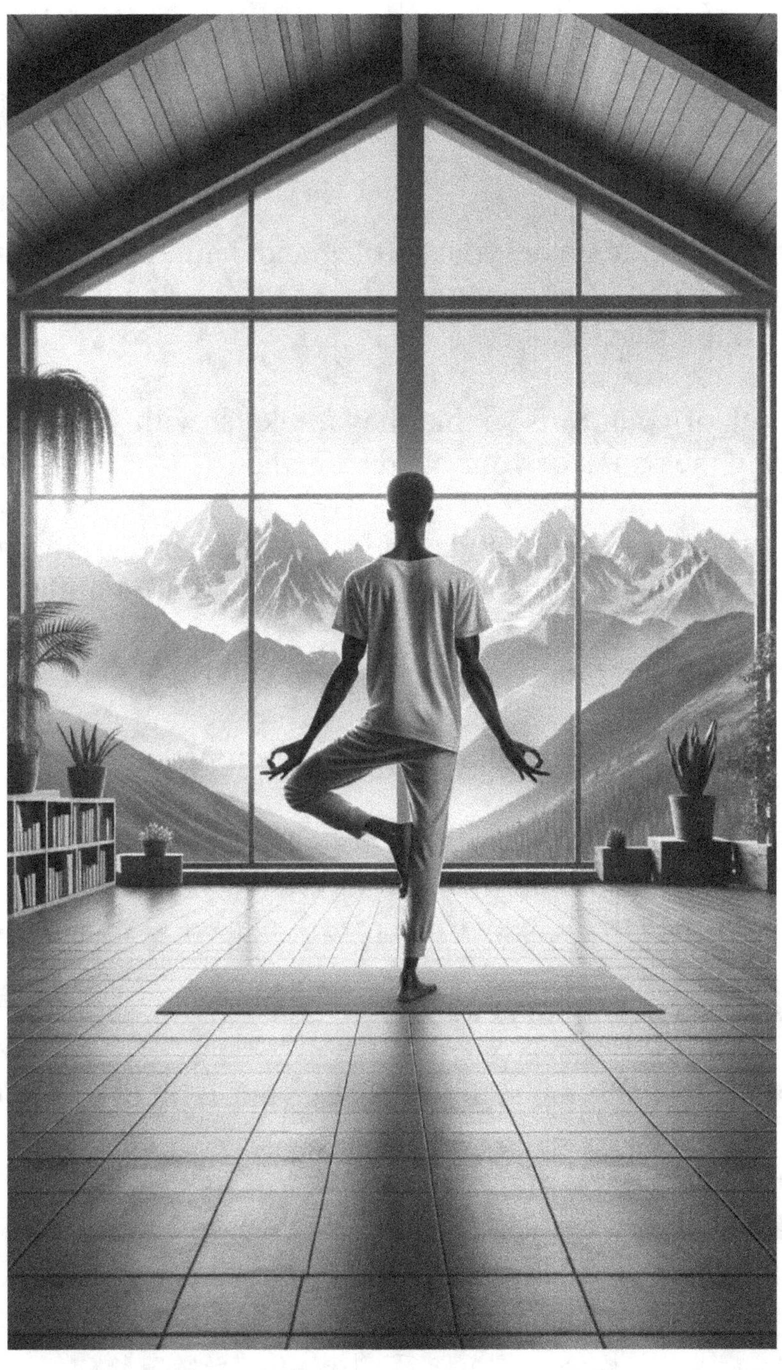

Pose of the Eagle

Eagle Pose is beneficial for both the suppleness and stability of the joints. This stance can help you become more aware of your body and its capabilities.

How it works:

Take a seat on a chair and bring your feet together, putting your hands on your thighs for support.

Bring your right leg over your left leg and behind you, bending your right knee as you go so that your right foot curls and stays on the right side of your left leg.

Raise both of your arms so that they are level with your shoulders and then bring the palms of your hands together.

Place the palms of your hands against each other by bringing the left hand beneath the right hand and then curling it around the right hand.

Hold this position for a count of thirty seconds.

On the other side, perform the identical actions.

Advantages:

Eagle Pose is a terrific way to increase your sense of self-awareness.

It helps one concentrate better.

It strengthens both your willpower and your faith in yourself.

Your leg muscles, all the way down to your feet, will get a workout from this stance.

It helps the digestive process.

Important things to keep in mind:

It is important to keep the elbows up. Maintain a straight line from your head to your shoulders.

It is important to note that individuals who have significant shoulder and arm issues should not attempt to perform this pose.

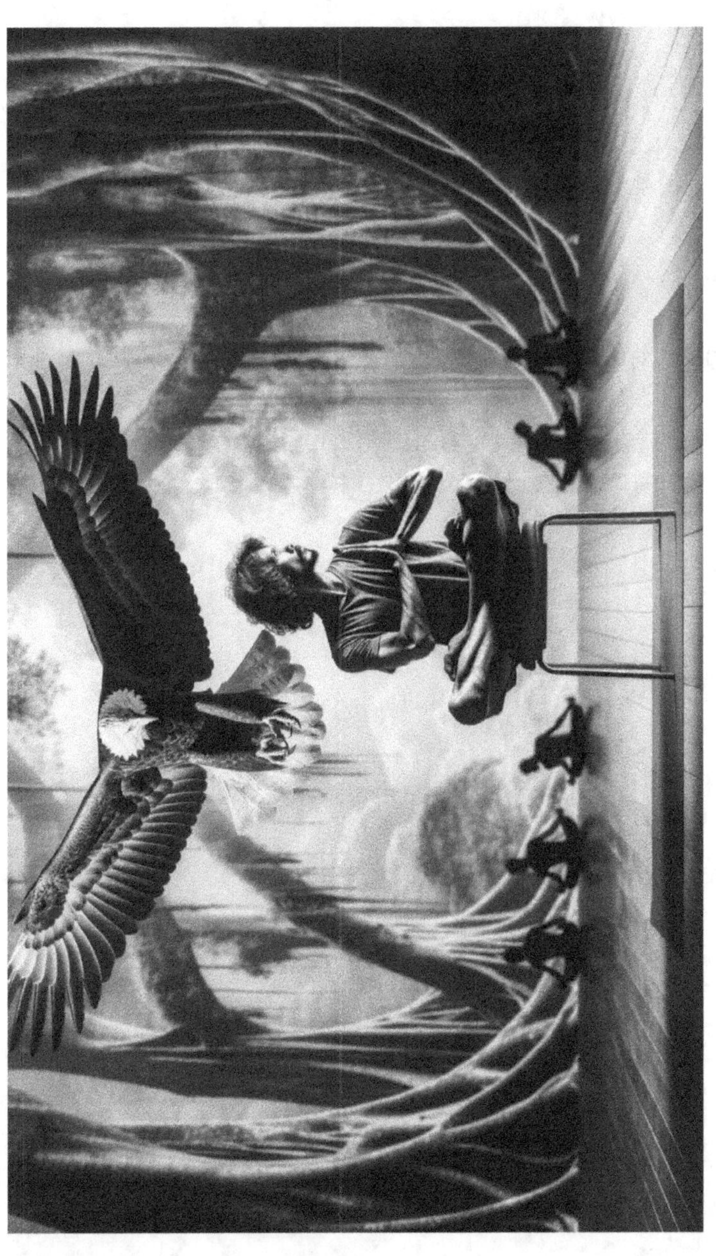

Arms with a Cow Face

Even though it might not look like it, the stance known as Cow Face Arms is an excellent method to relax and decompress. The tension in your shoulders and hands will melt away as a result.

How it works:

Place both feet in front of you while seated in a chair.

Raise your left palm by bringing your left hand around behind your back, bending it at the elbow, and then raising it so that it is higher up.

Raise your right arm above your head and then lower it back down to your side.

Join your hands in a fist.

Hold this position for a count of thirty seconds.

On the other side, perform the identical actions.

Advantages: This exercise will tone your arms.

Shoulder, upper back, and arm tension are all reduced as a result of this.

It helps the digestive process.

Important things to keep in mind:

Maintain proximity to your ear with the arm that is elevated and keep the elbow of that arm pointing upward.

It is important to note that individuals who have serious shoulder difficulties should not attempt to practice this pose.

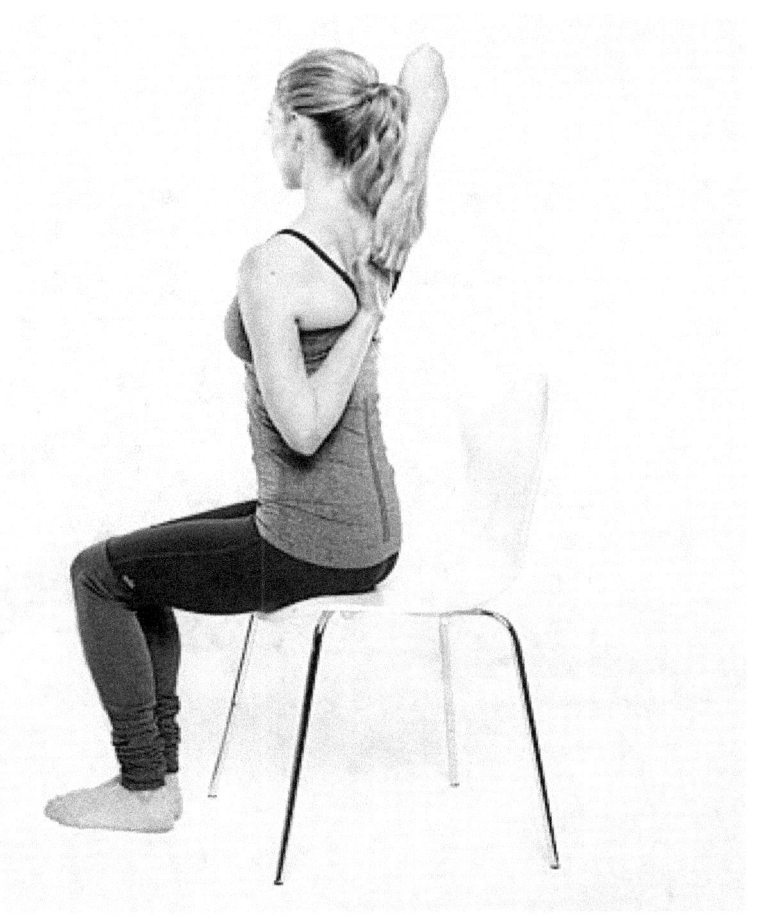

One of the most prevalent ailments experienced by many people, particularly those who are seated for lengthy periods of time at their desks at work, is soreness in the neck. Shoulder pain is another common ailment heard frequently. Arms are not an exception to this rule. The following are some straightforward workouts that can be carried out at any time. Muscle relaxation and stress reduction are two benefits that can be gained from performing these exercises while working.

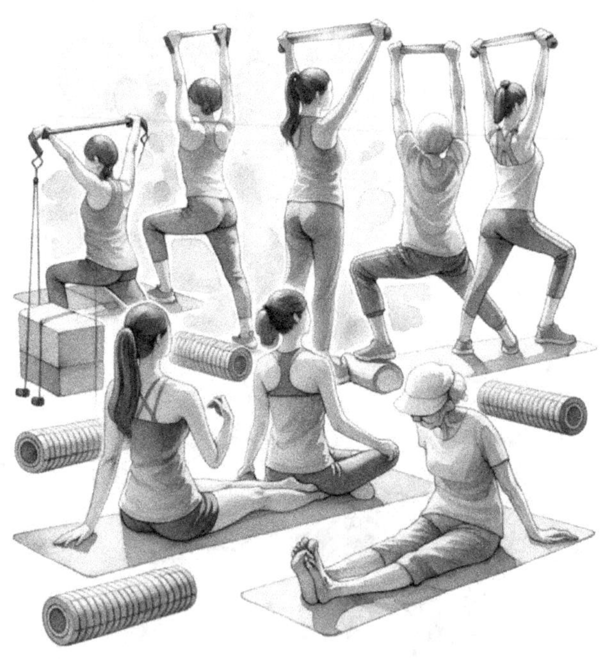

Flexibility can be increased by stretching your neck, which also helps to preserve the range of motion in your cervical joints. Regular practice of neck exercises can alleviate stiffness in the neck, which is a contributing factor in the development of neck discomfort.

Maintain a neutral spine when you are seated. Put as much of your chin as you can below your chest. Hold the position for a full five seconds. Keep your head tilted backwards for a full five seconds while holding the stance. It should be done five times.

Maintain good posture. Put a slight tilt of your head to the right. Keep the posture for a full three seconds. Come back to your starting position. Now turn your head in the other direction I just told you. Hold the posture for a total of three seconds. It should be done five times.

Maintain good posture. Relax your shoulders and look to the right while keeping your head turned in that direction. Hold this position for five seconds, then slowly turn your head to the left side of the room. After a countdown of 5 seconds, you should return to your normal position. It should be done five times.

Maintain good posture. Place the tip of your chin on the floor, then rotate your head to the right. Return to the starting position after rolling your neck to the left and backwards, then repeat the exercise. Perform the movement around the circle five times, then do it again going in the opposite direction, clockwise.

Exercises that focus on the shoulders can help alleviate discomfort and reduce shoulder stiffness. In addition to relieving discomfort in the upper arms, the stretches and exercises here can also assist relieve back pain. Working out your shoulders with exercises can assist improve the range of motion in your shoulders.

Raise your shoulders as high as you can and then slowly bring them back down. It should be done ten times.

If you are sitting, you should rest your arms on top of your thighs. You can relax the tension in your shoulders and let your arms hang at your sides if you perform the following exercise while standing. Put some pressure behind your shoulders, and then elevate them up toward the ceiling. Now, bring them in front of you and lower them. After finishing the movement in a clockwise manner, you will have completed a circular movement. Perform the action five times, then continue doing it in a direction that is counterclockwise.

Sideways, at the level of your shoulders, stretch your arms out. Without reducing the height of your body, bring your arms forward until the palms of your hands contact each other. Come back to your spot. Repeat the step ten times.

Swings of the Arm

Pain in the arms can be alleviated by performing arm swings. They increase your blood circulation while also toning your hands. Shoulder strength can also be improved with arm swings.

Raise the right arm forward and upward in a straight line. As you elevate your left arm, bring it back into position while you are doing so. Perform the same moves over and over again until you have finished all ten rounds.

You will complete the movement by reaching your right arm forward, bringing it up, and then bringing it behind you. Perform the action five times, then carry it out in reverse. Conduct the same action using your left hand.

The final word

The ancient practice of yoga has been adopted all over the Western world as a contemporary emblem of wellness, tranquility, and calm. This mind-body technique has received a lot of attention for its effectiveness in lowering stress and improving one's overall health and happiness. This ancient knowledge also offers a wide variety of benefits for one's physical health, which can compete with those offered by other types of activities. Although I am not one to make comparisons by nature, I think we can all agree that there are pros and cons to every type of physical activity. For example, because it is a low-impact form of exercise, yoga has more benefits than any other sports activity. It can eliminate, on every level, the benefits that come with going out at a gym.

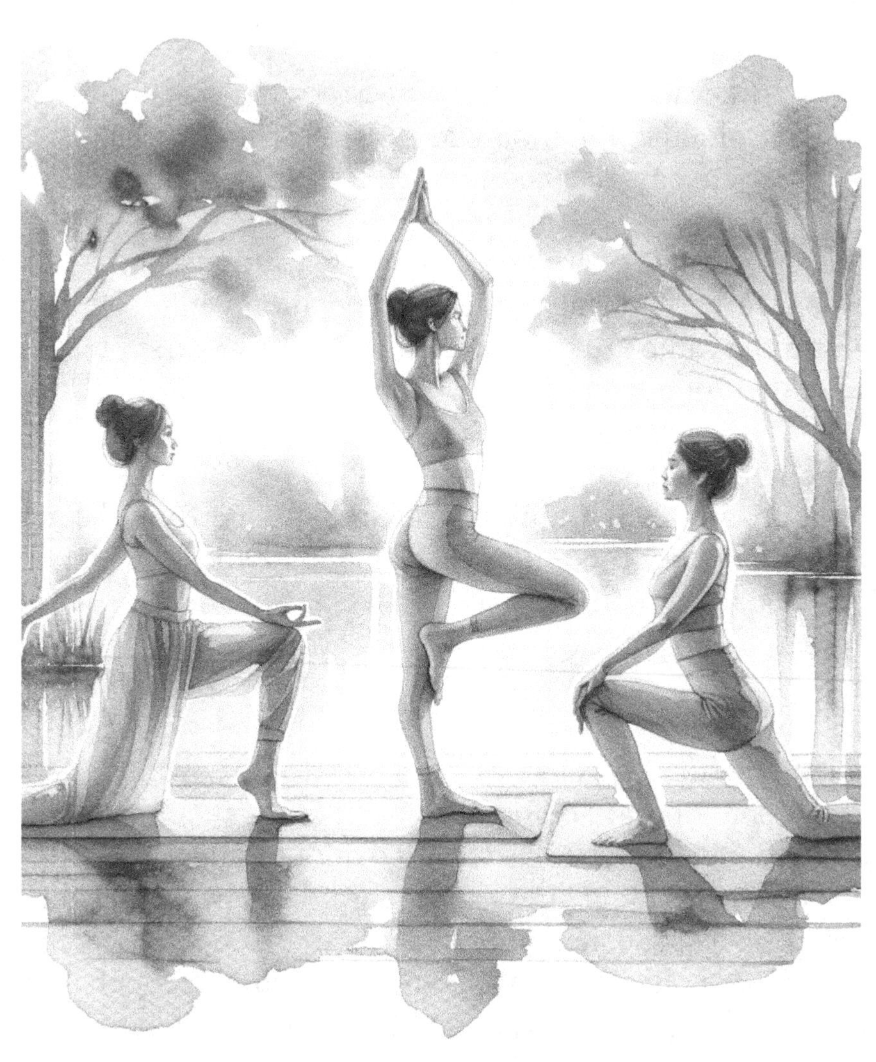

REMEMBER:
YOGA CAN BRING MANY BENEFITS TO YOUR LIFE!